PRENTICE HALL

HEART AND LUNG SOUNDS

WORKBOOK

PRENTICE HALL

HEART AND LUNG SOUNDS

WORKBOOK

JO ANNE CARRICK

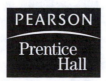

PEARSON

Prentice Hall

Upper Saddle River, New Jersey 07458

Notice: Care has been taken to confirm the accuracy of information presented in this book. The authors, editors, and the publisher, however, cannot accept any responsibility for errors or omissions or for consequences from application of the information in this book and make no warranty, express or implied, with respect to its contents.

The authors and publisher have exerted every effort to ensure that drug selections and dosages set forth in this text are in accord with current recommendations and practice at the time of publication. However, in view of ongoing research, changes in government regulations, and the constant flow of information relating to drug therapy and drug reactions, the reader is urged to check the package inserts of all drugs for any change in indications of dosage and for added warnings and precautions. This is particularly important when the recommended agent is a new and/or infrequently employed drug.

Publisher: Julie Levin Alexander
Publisher's Assistant: Regina Bruno
Editor-in-Chief: Maura Connor
Acquisitions Editor: Pamela Fuller
Associate Editor: Michael Giacobbe
Editorial Assistant: Melisa Baez
Director of Manufacturing and Production: Bruce Johnson
Managing Production Editor: Patrick Walsh
Production Liaison: Cathy O'Connell
Production Editor: Lindsey Hancock, Carlisle Publisher's Services, Inc.
Manufacturing Manager: Ilene Sanford
Manufacturing Buyer: Pat Brown
Design Director: Maria Guglielmo Walsh
Director of Marketing: Karen Allman
Senior Marketing Manager: Francisco Del Castillo
Marketing Coordinator: Michael Sirinides
Marketing Assistant: Patricia Linard
Media Editor: John Jordan
Media Production Manager: Amy Peltier
Media Project Manager: Tina Rudowski
Composition: Carlisle Publisher's Services, Inc.
Printer/Binder: Bind Rite Graphics
Cover Printer: Phoenix Color

Pearson Education Ltd.   Pearson Education Australia PTY, Limited
Pearson Education Singapore, Pte. Ltd.   Pearson Education North Asia Ltd.
Pearson Education Canada, Ltd.   Pearson Educación de Mexico, S.A. de C.V.
Pearson Education—Japan   Pearson Education Malaysia, Pte. Ltd.
                                           Pearson Education, Upper Saddle River, New Jersey

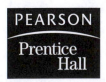

10 9 8 7 6 5 4 3 2 1
ISBN: 0-13-194901-2

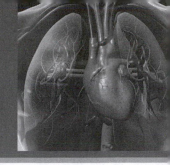

CONTENTS

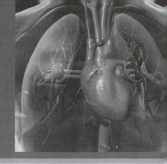

PRENTICE HALL *HEART AND LUNG SOUNDS* WORKBOOK

GETTING STARTED

This workbook is designed to help you successfully complete the *Prentice Hall Heart and Lung Sounds* CD, the independent study of heart and lung sounds. The workbook follows the content presented in the *Prentice Hall Heart and Lung Sounds* CD. The multimedia CD presents key concepts of physical assessment that are useful in the clinical management of clients with cardiopulmonary problems. After working your way through the *Prentice Hall Heart and Lung Sounds* CD and workbook, you will have a solid foundation on which to base your assessment of clients with cardiopulmonary disease. The CD and workbook will also help you if you are a practicing nurse with more advanced training who wants to brush up on concepts that are already in your knowledge base.

Follow the sections of the workbook as you navigate through the CD, reviewing the auditory and visual displays of heart and lung sounds. This workbook also contains activities and exercises using illustrations of heart and lung anatomy, exercises to reinforce your recognition of heart and lung sounds when reviewing the audio content found in the CD, and exercises to help build your knowledge base of key terms. At the end of the workbook you can test your ability to apply this information to real-life clinical situations. The questions are formatted as NCLEX® or Nursing Specialty Certification questions.

TIPS FOR LISTENING TO THE CD AND COMPLETING THE WORKBOOK

The *Prentice Hall Heart and Lung Sounds* CD and workbook can teach you how to recognize and differentiate between normal and abnormal heart and lung sounds. To get the most out of your experience, follow these steps:

1. Go through the CD—read the descriptions and listen to the audio portions one section at a time. The CD is divided into four sections, and you'll want to go through each: the Introduction, Common Heart Sounds, Common Lung Sounds, and Lung Sound Patterns.
2. After each section of the CD, use the workbook exercises to review and reinforce your knowledge of the content covered in that section.
3. When you have completed Sections 2 through 4 of the CD, take the audio quizzes to test your knowledge in recognizing normal and abnormal heart and lung sounds. You can repeat the quizzes several times until you can easily recognize the heart and lung sounds. Reviewing the corresponding workbook sections will help strengthen your understanding of what you are hearing.
4. The final section of the workbook consists of NCLEX®-style exam questions, designed to integrate the information as it relates to real clinical situations. After you've completed the CD and workbook review, test yourself by answering these questions. Answers are provided in the back of the workbook.

CHAPTER 1

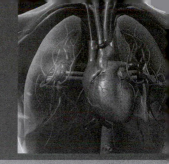

INTRODUCTION

THE CIRCULATORY SYSTEM

The heart, as the center of the circulatory system, is a major organ that controls the blood flow throughout the body. As blood passes through the chambers of the heart the physiologic mechanisms of the cardiac cycle create the movements of the heart muscle and valves that generate the heart sounds and assure perfusion of the coronary arteries and circulation to the rest of the body. As you complete your studies of the heart anatomy and heart sounds it is helpful to familiarize yourself with the anatomical structures of the heart, coronary blood flow, and the cardiac cycle. See Figures 1-1 and 1-2.

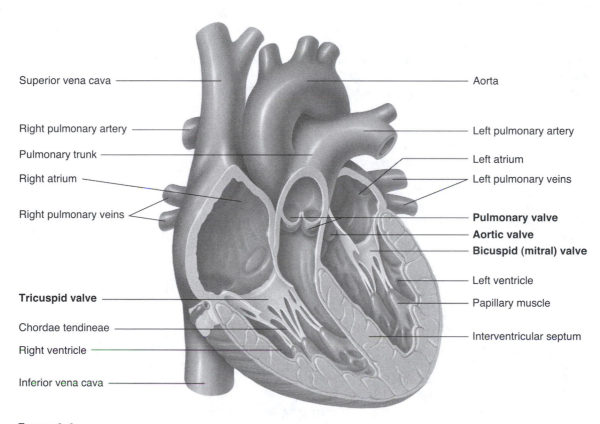

Superior vena cava

Right pulmonary artery

Pulmonary trunk

Right atrium

Right pulmonary veins

Tricuspid valve

Chordae tendineae

Right ventricle

Inferior vena cava

Aorta

Left pulmonary artery

Left atrium

Left pulmonary veins

Pulmonary valve

Aortic valve

Bicuspid (mitral) valve

Left ventricle

Papillary muscle

Interventricular septum

FIGURE 1-1
Anatomical structures of the heart chambers and valves.

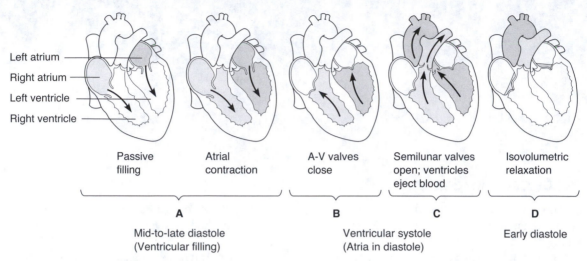

Left atrium

Right atrium

Left ventricle

Right ventricle

| Passive filling | Atrial contraction | A-V valves close | Semilunar valves open; ventricles eject blood | Isovolumetric relaxation |

A

Mid-to-late diastole
(Ventricular filling)

B

C

Ventricular systole
(Atria in diastole)

D

Early diastole

FIGURE 1-2
The opening and closing of the heart valves during the cardiac cycle.

CORONARY BLOOD FLOW

The main coronary arteries are located on the epicardium and branch across the cardiac muscle. Coronary perfusion occurs during diastole after the closure of the aortic valve and is regulated by aortic pressure. Review Figure 1-3 of coronary circulation and Table 1-1 that describe the location of the coronary arteries, the anatomical region of the heart that the artery supplies, the corresponding lead in the electrocardiogram, and clinical implications when damage to the heart muscle occurs with cardiac disease.

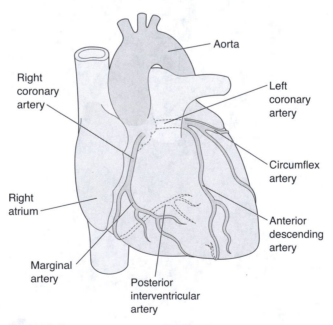

Aorta

Right coronary artery

Left coronary artery

Circumflex artery

Right atrium

Anterior descending artery

Marginal artery

Posterior interventricular artery

FIGURE 1-3
Coronary arterial circulation.

TABLE 1-1
Anatomical regions of the myocardium and their corresponding leads.

Anatomical Region	Coronary Artery	ECG Leads	Clinical Implications
Anteroseptal wall	LAD	V1, V2, V3, V4	Potential for significant muscle damage leading to pump failure and shock. Septal necrosis can lead to prolonged *PR* interval and heart block.
Left lateral wall	LCX	I, aVL, V5, V6	Some muscle damage and possible arrhythmias secondary to sinoatrial nodal dysfunction.
Inferior wall	RCA, LCX	II, III, aVF	Inferior wall infarctions result from occlusion of the RCA in about 80% of the cases and LCX in 20% of the cases. *ST* elevation greater in lead III than II suggests RCA, whereas *ST* elevation greater in lead II than III suggests LCX occlusion.
Right ventricular infarction	RCA	V4ᴿ, *ST* elevation in V1, II, III, aVF	Requires increased preload. Use of nitrates may be contraindicated.
Posterior wall	RCA	Tall *R* wave and *ST* depression in right precordial leads V1 and V2. V7 to V9 *ST* elevation.	

Adapted from Morton, P. G. (1996). Using the 12-lead ECG to detect ischemia, injury, and infarction. Critical Care Nurse, 16(2), 85–95.

EXERCISES

INSTRUCTIONS

Complete the following exercises after reviewing the introduction section of *A Simplified Introduction to Heart and Lung Sounds* CD.

Exercise #1 Heart Anatomy and Auscultatory Sites

Fill in the blanks to review the basic anatomy of the heart.

Heart Anatomy

The four cardiac valves are classified into two types—the (1) _____ [mitral and tricuspid] and the (2) _____ [aortic and pulmonic] valves. This is an important distinction. During systole, (3) _____ valves are closed and (4) _____ valves are open.

The Heart in Systole

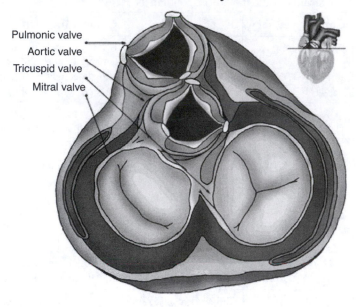

Pulmonic valve
Aortic valve
Tricuspid valve
Mitral valve

In diastole the opposite is true. (5) _____ valves are open to allow ventricular filling and (6) _____ valves are closed to prevent backflow of blood to the heart from either systemic circulation or pulmonary circulation.

The Heart in Diastole

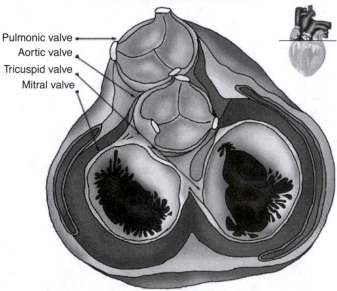

Pulmonic valve
Aortic valve
Tricuspid valve
Mitral valve

In normal persons these valves perform these functions very well. In disease the most common abnormalities of these valves are:

- Stenosis (narrowing)
- Insufficiency (failure to close completely—causing backflow or leaks, also known as regurgitation)
- A combination of stenosis and insufficiency

Exercise #2 Valvular Disease and Murmur Location

Complete the table with the type of heart valve condition indicating if there is stenosis or insufficiency of the valve.

Valve	Systolic Murmur	Diastolic Murmur
Aortic		
Pulmonic		
Mitral		
Tricuspid		

Exercise #3 Auscultatory Sites

There are four important areas used for listening to heart sounds. These are: aortic area, pulmonic area, tricuspid area, and mitral area (apex).

Label the sites of valve auscultation and the location of valves in the diagram below.

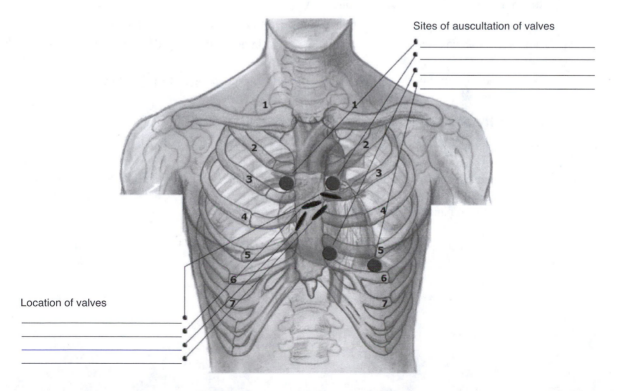

Sites of auscultation of valves

Location of valves

Exercise #4 Murmur Mechanism Guide

Complete the following matching quiz to help you identify the primary heart murmurs and their corresponding heart defect.

Murmur Mechanism Guide

1. Mitral stenosis
2. Atrial septal defect
3. Pulmonic regurgitation
4. Normal systole
5. Tricuspid regurgitation
6. Pulmonic stenosis
7. Aortic stenosis
8. Mitral regurgitation
9. Aortic insufficiency
10. Ventricular septal defect
11. Normal diastole
12. Tricuspid stenosis
13. Patent ductus arteriosis

_____ Turbulence caused by the flow of blood through a narrowed semilunar valve that radiates to the carotids

_____ Heard in the left sternal border, it results from backflow of the semilunar valve carrying unoxygenated blood

_____ Atrioventricular valves open and semilunar valves closed

_____ A continual connection between the aorta and pulmonary artery causing a pressure differential that results in continuous turbulence and a systolic murmur

_____ Flow of blood from a higher pressure chamber to the lower pressure; murmur is holosystolic

_____ Turbulence caused by a narrowed valve causing a diastolic murmur

_____ Caused by backflow of oxygenated blood during diastole

_____ Systolic murmur that may radiate to the axilla

_____ Mid-diastolic rumble due to increased blood flow through the tricuspid valve

_____ Atrioventricular valves closed, semilunar valves open

_____ Turbulent blood flow that the murmur may radiate to the apex via papillary muscles

_____ Narrowed valve with the murmur heard at the second intercostal space to the left of the sternal border

_____ Narrowed atrioventricular valve heard at the fifth intercostal space to the left of the sternal border

THE RESPIRATORY SYSTEM AND PULMONARY GAS EXCHANGE

The lungs are the central organ of the respiratory system whose primary function is the exchange of oxygen and carbon dioxide. As air passes through the upper airways to the lower airways it enters into the lung where a complex system of gas exchange occurs with the perfusion of the lung tissue by the pulmonary circulation. Interconnected with the cardiovascular system and the cardiac cycle, unoxygenated blood is circulated to the lung alveoli where gas exchange occurs. See Figure 1-4.

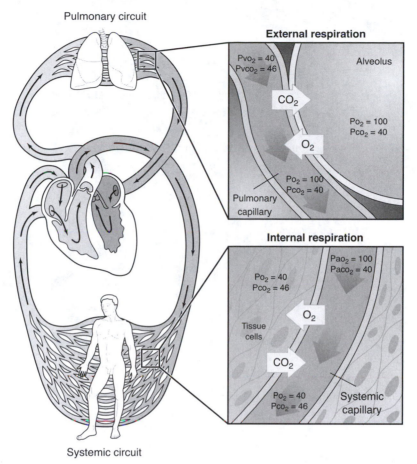

Pulmonary circuit

External respiration

$Pvo_2 = 40$
$Pvco_2 = 46$

Alveolus

CO_2

O_2

$Po_2 = 100$
$Pco_2 = 40$

$Po_2 = 100$
$Pco_2 = 40$

Pulmonary
capillary

Internal respiration

$Pao_2 = 100$
$Paco_2 = 40$

$Po_2 = 40$
$Pco_2 = 46$

O_2

Tissue
cells

CO_2

$Po_2 = 40$
$Pco_2 = 46$

Systemic
capillary

Systemic circuit

FIGURE 1-4
Cardiopulmonary circuit and respiration.

Pulmonary disease at any point in this process can interfere with the passage of air, effective gas exchange, and the transfer of oxygen necessary for all organ function and survival. Figure 1-5 illustrates the anatomy of the respiratory system. Note that the upper airways include the nasal cavity, the pharynx, and the larynx which provide an entrance for air into the lung. Any interference with these passages will interfere with the delivery of oxygen. If blocked, the sounds of the air movement across these chambers will change.

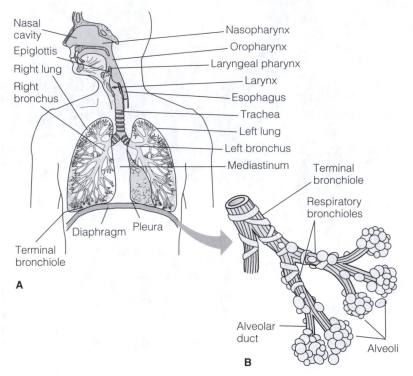

FIGURE 1-5
Anatomy of the respiratory system.

The lower airway structures include the trachea, bronchi, bronchioles, and alveoli. These structures may be affected by disease processes that not only obstruct the flow of air but also affect gas exchange at the microscopic level. In addition, disease conditions of the pleura, diaphragm, and intercostal muscles will alter respiration and gas exchange.

The end result from disease is the lack of oxygen in the blood. As oxygenated blood moves through the pulmonary capillaries, it meets with the alveoli for exchange of oxygen. If lung tissue is damaged blood is shunted past the alveoli without oxygenation. This can occur due to anatomical shunts with heart and lung problems such as ventricular septal defects. Other shunts include capillary shunts seen with alveolar collapse and consolidation and shuntlike effects from decreased ventilation and diffusion effects seen in high-acuity patients. Figure 1-6 illustrates the types of physiologic shunts.

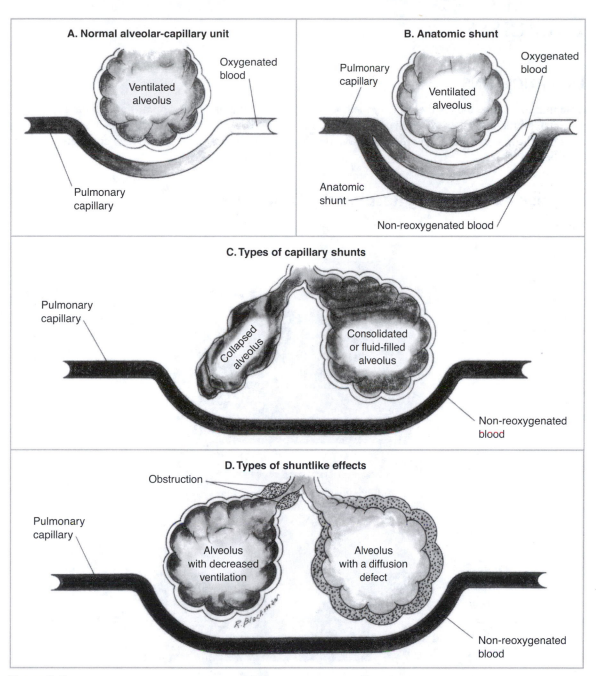

FIGURE 1-6
Types of physiologic shunt.

EXERCISES

INSTRUCTIONS

Listening to lung sounds is the primary method used to assess the movement of air through the respiratory system. Completing the exercises in the workbook and the CD will take you through a guided process to learn how to identify normal and abnormal lung sounds. Begin by listening to the CD and then complete the exercises below.

Exercise #5 Assessing Respiratory Function

Label the structures of the lung anatomy.

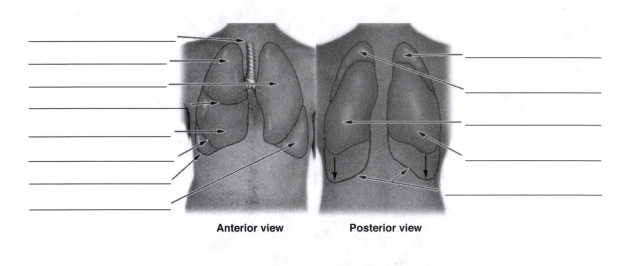

Anterior view   **Posterior view**

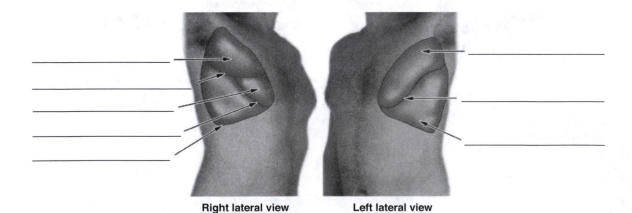

Right lateral view   **Left lateral view**

Exercise #6 Auscultatory Sites for Lung Sounds

The trachea or windpipe branches at the level of the second rib into two smaller airways: the right and left main stem bronchi. These then enter the lung. The right main stem bronchus branches to supply the upper, middle, and lower lobes of the right lung. The left main stem bronchus divides into smaller bronchi, which lead to the upper and lower lobes.

The figure below identifies the recommended sites for auscultation. These are a minimum for a routine examination of a patient with no known pulmonary problems. When respiratory disease is present, you may need to listen at more sites.

Fill in the boxes with the corresponding anatomical part.

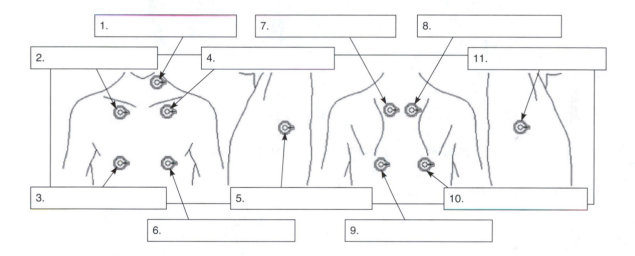

Physical Assessment of the Respiratory System in the Client with Respiratory Disease

Physical assessment of the respiratory system is extremely important for the proper management of patients. This may seem surprising at a time when we have such technologically superior diagnostic techniques, such as CT scans, pulmonary arteriograms, and MRIs. There are times when proper knowledge of physical assessment can be lifesaving. This includes detection of a collapsed lung, upper airway obstruction due to a foreign body, adequacy of the oxygen supply, and pleural effusions. But even in the routine assessment of patients, the knowledge gained from physical assessment is often what guides management of patients and the ordering of additional tests. This section will concentrate on the parts of physical assessment that are important in most common situations; that is, in routine practice.

Physical assessment is divided into four categories: inspection, palpation, percussion, and auscultation. The content in the CD will focus on percussion and auscultation. The following learning activity focuses on percussion. Auscultation will be covered in the sections discussing normal and abnormal lung sounds.

Percussion

Percussion involves tapping the chest to determine its resonance. *(The method was invented by Auggen-bruegger over 200 years ago. Auggenbruegger was a wine merchant's son. He used the skills learned from his father in detecting the fullness of a wine keg to detect fluid in the lungs of his patients.)*

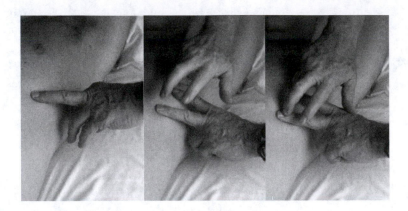

Percussion is performed by a finger striking upon another finger as illustrated.

Exercise #7 Physical Assessment of the Respiratory System

1. What is the purpose of percussion? _____

_____

2. Define the difference in percussion pitch over the normal lung and over denser tissue.

_____

3. Fill in the categories in the table below:

Type of Resonance	Source of Sounds	Underlying Disease Pathology
Normal resonance		
Hyperresonance		
Decreased resonance		

4. It is recommended that you return to the CD to review the different resonance sounds. After reviewing the sounds, complete the study questions below.

    A. The location for percussion in the following figure denotes the anatomical site of the heart. What type of resonance sound would you expect to hear at this site? _____

    B. If the examiner was percussing on the patient's right side near rib 7, what type of resonance sound would you expect to hear? _____

    C. What organ would contribute to the characteristic sound? _____

    D. The percussion note is _____ during inspiration as the diaphragm moves downward and the lung fills with air.

    E. During expiration the percussion note changes to _____ as air moves out of the lung and the diaphragm moves upward to its resting position.

    F. List conditions where the diaphragm becomes paralyzed, thus eliminating the changes in percussion. _____

_____

_____

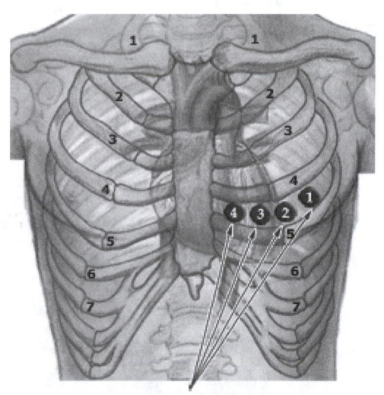

Percussion sites

CHAPTER 2

COMMON HEART SOUNDS

DIRECTIONS

The following exercises correspond with the second section of *A Simplified Introduction to Heart and Lung Sounds* CD. In this chapter you will study the components and defining characteristics of normal heart sounds, extra heart sounds, changes in heart rhythm, and murmurs. You should begin by reviewing the content on the CD, then proceed through the exercises in the workbook. You may want to refer back to the CD to complete the exercises and enhance the learning of the content.

NORMAL CHARACTERISTICS OF S1 AND S2

To listen to the normal heart sounds use the diaphragm of the stethoscope placed over the left chest just distal to the nipple. This is the location to best hear S1 and S2 and is the primary location for auscultation of the apical pulse. As noted in the following figure, you may move your stethoscope to the third intercostal space to auscultate S2, which will be louder in this area. Review the following figure which shows the sites for auscultation of the heart valves. Answer the following questions that describe the normal characteristics of S1 and S2.

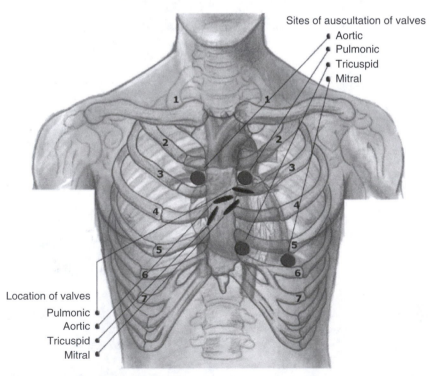

Complete the matching questions that follow.

EXERCISES

Exercise #1 Common Heart Sound Review

1. Closure of mitral and tricuspid valves
2. Closure of aortic and pulmonic valves
3. Ventricular ejection (systole)
4. Rising phase of pulse
5. Infant heart rates
6. Tachycardia
7. Athlete heart rates
8. Children age 1–10 years heart rates
9. Declining phase of pulse
10. Bradycardia
11. Children age 10 years and older heart rates
12. Lub
13. Ventricular filling (diastole)
14. Dub

_____ Start of systole

_____ S1 sound corresponds with this phase of the pulse

_____ S2 sound corresponds with this phase of the pulse

_____ Heart rate below normal values

_____ Time between the first and second heart sound

_____ 70–120 beats/minute

_____ End of systole

_____ 40–60 beats/minute

_____ Rate above normal values

_____ 100–160 beats/minute

_____ First heart sound

_____ 60–100 beats/minute

_____ Time between the second heart sound and the following first heart sound

_____ Second heart sound

CHARACTERISTICS OF S3 AND S4

S3 and S4 can occur in normal persons or be associated with pathological processes. Because of their cadence or rhythmic timing S3 and S4 are called gallops. Gallops are low frequency sounds, lower than both S1 and S2. It is best to listen to gallops with the bell of the stethoscope resting lightly on the skin. Pressing firmly with the bell often reduces transmission of gallops to below the hearing threshold. Review the content and sounds on _A Simplified Introduction to Heart and Lung Sounds_ CD, then complete the following questions and learning activities.

Exercise #2 Differentiating S3 and S4

Fill in the following table. This will help you identify the differences between S3 and S4 as well as the normal and pathological processes of both heart sounds.

Heart Sound	Associated Heart Process	Normal Characteristics	Pathologic Characteristics	Cadence Word Clue
S3				
S4				

IRREGULAR HEART RATE AND SPLITTING OF S1 AND S2

Heart rate variability and splitting of S1 and S2 will occur in the normal heart. However, as is the case with S3 and S4, pathologic conditions can cause changes in rate and rhythm and splitting of the first and second heart sound. It is recommended that you review the content presented in *A Simplified Introduction to Heart and Lung Sounds* CD prior to completing the learning activities that follow.

Exercise #3 Rate, Rhythm, and Splitting of Heart Sounds

Answer the following short answer essay questions.

1. Describe the changes in abdominal and intrathoracic pressure during inspiration and the effect it has on venous return. _____

   _____

   _____

2. How does the heart respond to the normal changes that occur with inspiration and expiration?

   _____

   _____

   _____

3. List a heart rhythm that may cause an irregular heart rate that is not associated with the respiratory cycle. How can you identify the cause? _____

   _____

   _____

   _____

   _____

4. If splitting of S1 occurs, what is the action that causes this sound?_____

   _____

5. If splitting of S2 occurs, what is the action that causes this sound?_____
_____
_____

6. Describe the changes in abdominal and intrathoracic pressure during inspiration and the effect this has on venous return and *its effect on the right heart.* _____
_____
_____
_____
_____

Exercise #4 Characteristics of Splitting of S2

Prolonged splitting of S2 is associated with heart disease such as atrial septal defect or right bundle branch block and may be normal in infants and children. Paradoxical splitting of the second heart sound, however, can occur. Complete the following table to help you differentiate the characteristics that occur with the splitting of S2.

Splitting of S2	Cause	Effect on the Heart Valves
Normal		
Mild Paradoxical		
Advanced Paradoxical		

Heart Murmurs

Exercise #5

Label the following figures describing the five mechanisms that generate heart murmur sounds.

1.

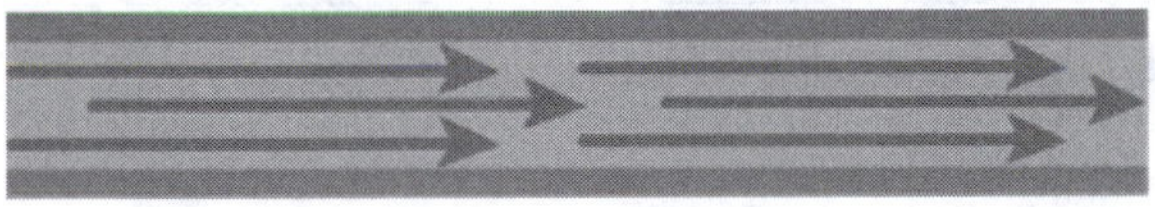

Cause: _____
_____

Clinical conditions in which murmur can occur:

_____

_____

2.

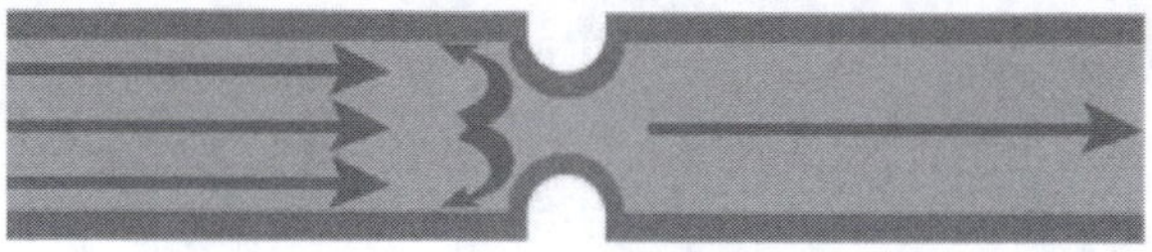

Cause: _____

_____

Clinical conditions in which murmur can occur:

_____

_____

3.

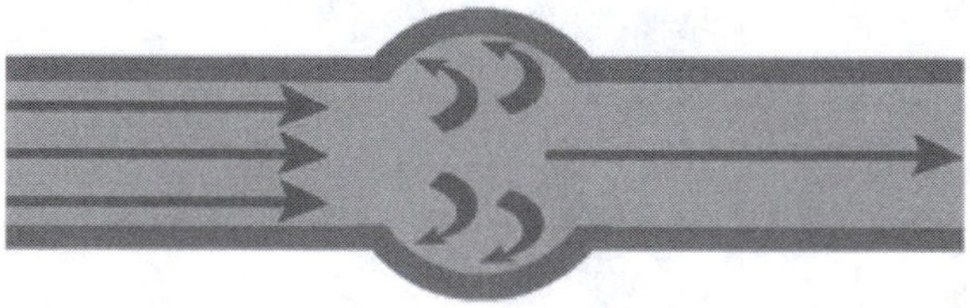

Cause: _____

_____

Clinical conditions in which murmur can occur:

_____

_____

4.

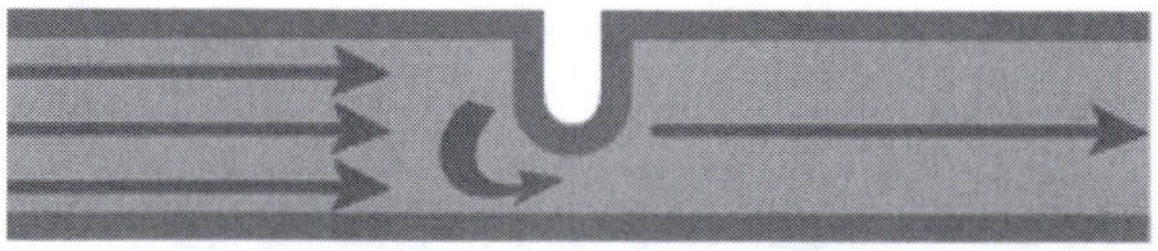

Cause: _____

_____

Clinical conditions in which murmur can occur:

_____

_____

5.

Cause: _____

_____

Clinical conditions in which murmur can occur:

_____

_____

CARDIAC MURMUR ASSESSMENT

Cardiac murmur assessment is based on their timing in the cardiac cycle, as well as their shape, location and radiation, pitch, intensity, and duration. The following exercises will help you synthesize the information presented in *A Simplified Introduction to Heart and Lung Sounds* CD so that you can become familiar with the terminology used to characterize murmurs.

Exercise #6 Murmur Timing

Answer the following questions:

1. Murmurs heard during systole are referred to as _____ murmurs.

2. Murmurs always associated with pathological conditions are_____ murmurs.

3. What condition would make it difficult to determine murmur timing and why?_____

_____

4. A method to confirm whether the murmur is systolic or diastolic is to confirm systole by: _____.

_____

5. _____ murmurs are heard in both systole and diastole.

6. Define "to and fro" murmurs._____

_____

Exercise #7 Murmur Location and Radiation

Murmur location and radiation will correspond with murmur pathophysiology. Mark the following figure to indicate the best location for the following heart valve diseases. You may want to refer to the Murmur Mechanism Guide for answers.

- Aortic insufficiency
- Aortic stenosis

■ Pulmonic regurgitation
■ Pulmonic stenosis
■ Tricuspid stenosis
■ Tricuspid regurgitation
■ Mitral stenosis
■ Mitral regurgitation

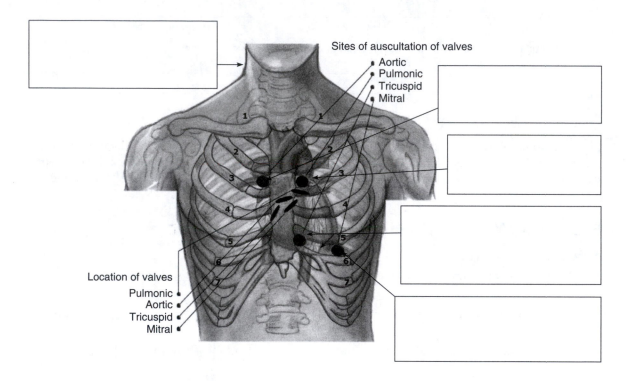

Exercise #8 Murmur Grading

Complete the following matching exercise that classifies murmurs according to intensity or grade.

Murmur Grading

1. Grade 1   4. Grade 4
2. Grade 2   5. Grade 5
3. Grade 3   6. Grade 6

_____ Loud murmur; a thrill may be present

_____ Faint murmur that can only be heard after a few seconds

_____ Loud murmur that can be heard with the chest piece just removed from and not touching the skin; a thrill is present

_____ Faint murmur that is heard immediately

_____ Loud murmur that can be heard if only the edge of the stethoscope is in contact with the skin; a thrill is present

_____ Moderate murmur intensity

Exercise #9 Murmur Shape

Define the murmur shape in the following figures and complete the corresponding questions.

_____

_____

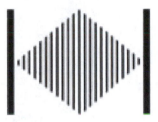

Crescendo/Decrescendo—

1. What are the primary causes of this type of murmur shape? _____

_____

2. What are other names for this type of murmur?_____

_____

Holosystolic—

1. What is another name for this type of murmur shape?_____

_____

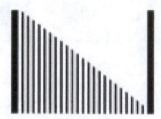

Decrescendo—

1. What type of murmur shows this characteristic shape? _____

   _____

2. How does the turbulence in blood flow from this type of murmur cause the characteristic sound?

   _____

   _____

Exercise #10 Systolic and Diastolic Murmur Timing

Systolic and diastolic murmurs can be described in terms of intensity and timing. This is either early, mid, or late and will correspond with their presence in relation to S1 and S2. Complete the following table to help you differentiate these unique characteristics of systolic and diastolic murmurs' timing.

Type of Murmur	Timing	Other Defining Characteristics
Early Systolic		
Mid Systolic		
Late Systolic		
Early Diastolic		

Type of Murmur	Timing	Other Defining Characteristics
Mild Diastolic		
Late Diastolic		

Exercise #11 Systolic Murmur Pitch

Another characteristic is the pitch of a murmur that is affected by pressure gradients. The pitch will be higher over a stenotic aortic valve than over a stenotic mitral valve.

    1. Explain why this occurs._____

_____

_____

DEVELOPING AN INTEGRATED TECHNIQUE FOR LISTENING TO HEART SOUNDS

The Events of the Cardiac Cycle

The cardiac cycle is a combination of many events reflective of its unique physiological process. As electrical activity moves through the heart, the cardiac muscle responds with the stages of depolarization, repolarization, contraction, and relaxation. Blood flows through the heart chambers creating pressure that results in the opening and closing of valves. This allows the blood to travel through the pulmonary and systemic circuits.

    When listening to the heart sounds, it is important to view the assessment as an integrated process of the cardiac cycle. The following exercises are designed to aid in identifying the components of the cardiac cycle as they are reflected by the heart sounds and other aspects of cardiac circulation.

Exercise #12 Electrocardiogram

The electrocardiogram tracing is a reflection of the depolarization/repolarization of the cardiac muscle. The P wave corresponds with atrial depolarization. The QRS complex is the result of ventricular depolarization across the ventricular musculature which results in ventricular contraction. The last wave is the T wave which is the repolarization of the ventricles. The shape of the electrocardiogram waveform will vary based on the lead the pattern is viewed from and any associated disease. For the purpose of this discussion and exercise, we will use a normal electrocardiogram pattern in the primary lead II view. This is the common lead that is used when the patient is placed on cardiac monitoring. The tracing that follows is a representation of the EKG (electrocardiogram) in lead II.

In the Following Figure:

1. In Figure 2-1, fill in the boxes on the electrocardiogram tracing that correspond with the waveforms and physiologic response to an electrical stimulus on the heart muscle. All of the following points must be labeled:

    P wave, QRS wave, T wave

    Atrial depolarization

    Ventricular depolarization/contraction

    Ventricular repolarization/relaxation

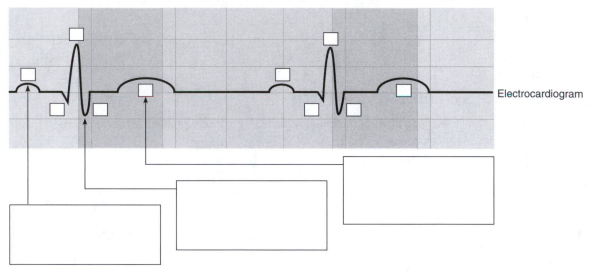

Electrocardiogram

FIGURE 2-1

Exercise #13 Phonocardiogram

The phonocardiogram is a tracing of the heart sounds associated with the electrocardiogram. During the cardiac cycle, valves open and close to create the heart sounds, creating the normal cardiac sounds of S1 and S2. Sometimes normally and often when disease is present, additional heart sounds are heard during the cardiac cycle. These sounds are the S3 and S4 heart sounds. As you work through exercises in this book and complete the activities of *A Simplified Introduction to Heart and Lung Sounds* CD, you will develop skill in the recognition of the various normal and abnormal heart sounds. The heart sounds can be plotted along the EKG tracing as a way to show where they occur in the cardiac cycle.

   S1 marks the beginning of systole and the closing of the atrioventricular valves. S2 marks the beginning of diastole and the closure of the semilunar (aortic and pulmonary) valves. S3 is heard in early diastole and S4 is heard in late diastole. Complete the following exercise to plot these sounds and the phases of the cardiac cycle.

In Figure 2-2:

1. Mark the systolic and diastolic phases of the cardiac cycle.

2. Mark the location of S1 and S2 on the EKG tracing as they correspond with the phases of the cardiac cycle.

3. Mark the location of where S3 and S4 occur on the EKG tracing as they correspond with the phases of the cardiac cycle.

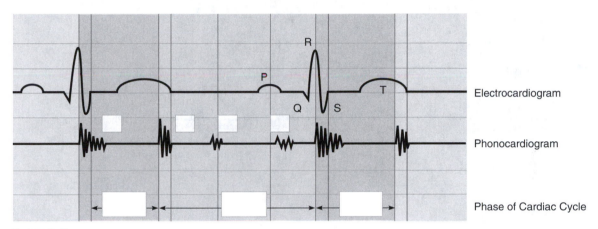

FIGURE 2-2

Exercise #14 Ventricular Volume/Pulse

As the ventricle contracts, blood is circulated through the body. This force causes a filling in the peripheral arteries that creates a palpable pulse. A technique to help the clinician identify the heart sounds while listening to them is to palpate the radial or carotid pulse. During the upswing of the pulse, ventricular contraction, the first heart sound is heard. During the downswing of the pulse, ventricular relaxation, the second heart sound is heard. Using this technique is especially helpful in identifying heart sounds when the heart rate is fast. Complete the following exercise to help you identify the upswing and downswing of the pulse as it corresponds with the EKG tracing, phases of the cardiac cycle, and the occurrence of the heart sounds.

In Figure 2-3:

1. Mark the location of S1 and S2.

2. Mark the phases of the cardiac cycle.

3. Place an arrow beside the heart sound that indicates an upswing or downswing of the pulse as it occurs in the cardiac cycle.

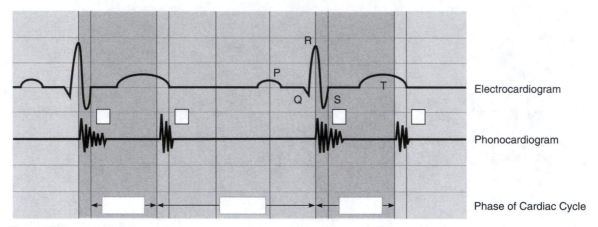

FIGURE 2-3

Exercise #15 Ventricular Volume, Atrial Pressure, Ventricular Pressure, and Aortic Pressure

Pressure waves can be plotted along the same pattern to correspond with the electrocardiogram tracing, the phonocardiogram, and the arterial pressure waveform. In critical care settings, the electrocardiogram and the atrial pressure waveform are common hemodynamic monitoring tools. Figure 2-4 illustrates the volume pressure effects occurring in the heart chambers during the cardiac cycle. To assist you in completing the exercise, the figure is divided into two phases. Answer the questions that are related to the events of the cardiac cycle.

Exercise #16 Phase 1 of the Cardiac Cycle

Complete the Following Fill-in-the-Blank Questions Related to Phase 1:

1. As ventricular volume increases, the atrioventricular valve _____. This creates the _____ heart sound of the cardiac cycle.

2. The closing of the A-V valve and ventricular _____ marks the beginning of the _____ phase of the cardiac cycle.

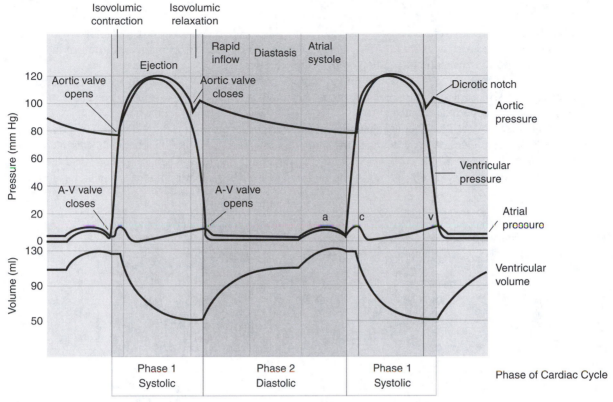

FIGURE 2-4

3. The corresponding waveform on the electrocardiogram is the _____.
4. Ventricular volume is at its highest at the beginning of this phase. As ventricular pressure increases, an _____ of the pulse is felt when palpated.

Exercise #17 Phase 2 of the Cardiac Cycle

Complete the Following Fill-in-the-Blank Questions Related to Phase 2:

1. As ventricular volume decreases, the aortic and pulmonary valves _____. This creates the _____ heart sound of the cardiac cycle.
2. The closing of the aortic and pulmonary valves and ventricular _____ marks the beginning of the _____ phase of the cardiac cycle.
3. The corresponding waveform on the electrocardiogram is the _____.
4. Ventricular volume is at its lowest at the beginning of this phase. As ventricular pressure decreases, a _____ of the pulse is felt when palpated.

SUMMARY

The events of the cardiac cycle are reflections of time, pressure, and volume. It also includes electrical activity through the heart, movement of blood through the heart chambers, and the opening and closing of the heart valves. Figure 2-5 illustrates the integration of all of these events.

Clinicians can monitor these activities through various assessment tools. They include electrocardiogram monitoring, invasive hemodynamic pressure monitoring, and the physical assessment of listening to heart sounds and palpating peripheral pulses.

In many disease conditions, subtle changes will occur requiring the clinician to be skillful in monitoring and assessment techniques. As you continue the study of normal and abnormal heart sounds presented in *A Simplified Introduction to Heart and Lung Sounds* CD turn to this diagram to help you understand the relationship of the sounds to basic physiology of the cardiac cycle and the integration of assessment techniques.

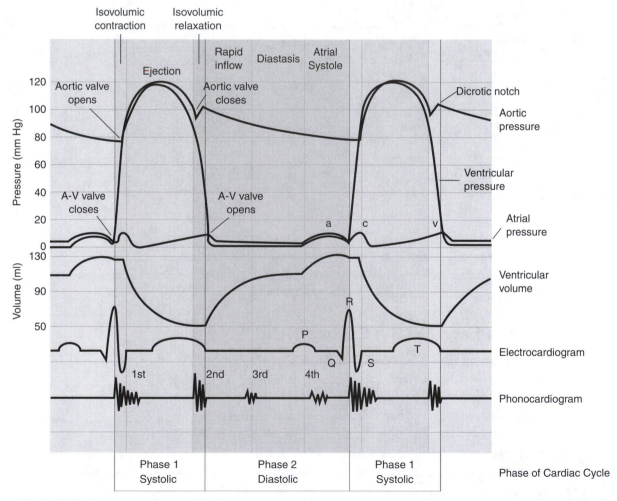

FIGURE 2-5

Reprinted from *Pathophysiology,* 3rd Edition, Copstead, L. C. and Banasik, J. L. Figure 17-6 page 436, 2005 with permission from Elsevier.

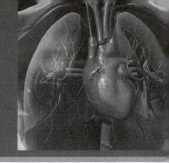

CHAPTER 3

COMMON LUNG SOUNDS

INSTRUCTIONS

Review the section of *A Simplified Introduction to Heart and Lung Sounds* CD which discusses common lung sounds. In that part of the CD you will review and listen to normal and abnormal or adventitious sounds. The CD and workbook exercises are designed to help reinforce the learning and assist you in developing competencies in the assessment of clients' normal and abnormal breath sounds.

Exercise #1 Normal Breathing Sounds

Answer the following short answer essay questions that discuss the characteristics of normal breath sounds.

1. Define the two types of breath sounds that can be heard through a stethoscope.

Normal: _____

_____

Adventitious: _____

_____

2. Normal breath sounds are heard and described. Normal breath sounds are both inspiratory and expiratory. They occur as the air moves in and out of the chest when a person breathes normally. There are two important types, bronchial and vesicular. The differences can be easily distinguished by listening to examples presented in *A Simplified Introduction to Heat and Lung Sounds* CD.

Place a V or a B next to the characteristic that matches the description of a vesicular or bronchial breath sound.

_____ Resemble wind moving through trees, causing leaves to rustle

_____ Heard over large airways

_____ Louder during expiration

_____ Air being blown through a cardboard roll

_____ Heard over the trachea or in the midline of the upper anterior chest

_____ Heard over the right upper anterior chest and on the back between the scapulae, both to the right and left of the sternum

_____ Heard over small airways of the chest

_____ When heard at the base of the lungs, are considered abnormal

_____ Commonly heard when lung tissue becomes solid

_____ Pneumonia, or any situation in which the alveoli and the small airways are filled with fluid, will produce these breath sounds in abnormal locations

_____ Heard louder on expiration than inspiration

_____ Heard louder on inspiration than expiration

Exercise #2 Sound Visualization

The exercises in this section are designed to assist you with understanding aspects of sound visualization. It is recommended that you complete these exercises while using the lung sound section of *A Simplified Introduction to Heart and Lung Sounds* CD.

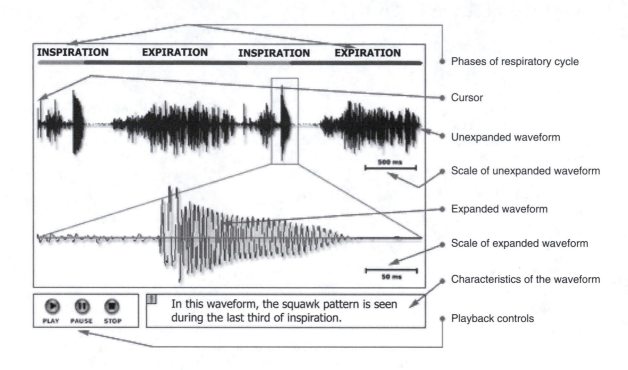

Answer the Following Questions:

1. Describe the differences between expanded and unexpanded waveforms.

    Expanded: _____

    _____

    _____

    _____

    Unexpanded: _____

    _____

    _____

    _____

2. Explain what amplitude–versus–time plots of typical lung sounds in an expanded time scale will

    show. _____

    _____

Exercise #3 Adventitious Sounds

Unexpected in normal persons, adventitious sounds are abnormal breath sounds that have various characteristics. The following workbook exercise is designed to help you understand the characteristics of the different adventitious breath sounds. Place the defining characteristics of the adventitious breath sounds as you listen to the different adventitious breath sounds in *A Simplified Introduction to Heart and Lung Sounds* CD. Once completed, this table may be a useful reference for you as you listen to the sound examples in the lung sound pattern section of *A Simplified Introduction to Heart and Lung Sounds* CD.

Adventitious Sound	Description	Acoustic Characteristic	Potential Sources of Abnormal Sound	Discontinuous vs. Continuous
Fine Crackles				
Coarse Crackles				
Wheezes				
Squawks				
Rhonchi				
Pleural Rub				
Stridor				

Exercise #4 Approach to the Patient

Review the following figure and answer the short answer essay questions that discuss how and where to listen to breath sounds.

Auscultatory sites for breath sounds:

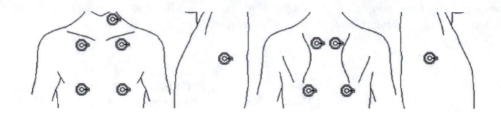

1. When approaching the patient to listen to breath sounds, how should the patient be instructed to breathe? _____

_____

_____

2. What would you instruct the client to do if he or she becomes dizzy during the exam? _____

_____

_____

3. Where should you begin the auscultatory exam of breath sounds?_____

_____

_____

4. What part of the stethoscope is used for auscultating breath sounds?_____

_____

_____

5. What physical feature on the patient may interfere while listening to breath sounds and resemble fine crackles?_____

_____

_____

6. What can be done to eliminate this problem?_____

_____

_____

7. In what part of the lung is the breath sound normally less intense?_____

_____

_____

CHAPTER 4

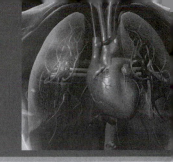

LUNG SOUND PATTERNS

Exercise #1 Lung Sound Analyzer

Fill-in-the-Blank

1. A multichannel lung sound analyzer is called a _____.

2. Following the recording of breath sounds, the lung sound analyzer computer will automatically
   calculate _____ and _____ and
   display their location on the chest wall as their timing in the respiratory cycle.

Exercise #2 Lung Sounds and Disease

Matching–Match the Disease Condition to the Lung Sound Characteristic Listed Below

1. Asthma
2. Congestive heart failure
3. Pneumonia
4. COPD

5. Bronchiectasis
6. Interstitial fibrosis
7. Tuberculosis
8. Pneumothorax

_____ Decreased, end-expiratory wheezing; rhonchi that clear with coughing and basilar crackles

_____ Numerous crackles over the chest from bases to apices

_____ Crackles are common over affected area, often over posterior bases, present for years without changing

_____ Crackles over affected region, dullness to percussion, decreased breath sounds and bronchial breathing

_____ Absence of breath sounds over affected area

_____ Fine crackles, squawks, and short wheezes

_____ Cardinal feature is wheezing

_____ Abnormal lung sounds heard in upper half of chest, inspiratory crackles, amphoric or cavernous sounds

Exercise #3 Changes in Lung Sound Pattern

True and False

_____ **1.** When wheezes cease and the chest is quiet this is an indication that the asthmatic is no longer at risk.

_____ **2.** In the patient with COPD, the inspiratory phase is prolonged.

_____ **3.** While crackles are present over the chest from bases to the apices in the congestive heart patient, in early stages, crackles may only be heard at the bases.

_____ **4.** Viral pneumonia may present with little or no auscultatory abnormalities.

_____ **5.** Patients with fibrotic changes are less likely to have crackles on auscultation if the fibrosis is due to interstitial pulmonary fibrosis rather than sarcoidosis.

_____ **6.** In the presence of pneumothorax, breath sounds on the other side may be decreased in intensity.

CHAPTER 5

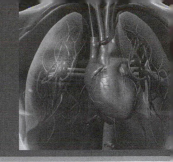

NCLEX®—CERTIFICATION QUESTIONS

1. The nurse is caring for a client who was admitted last night for shortness of breath. The client has a history of an acute MI and coronary artery bypass surgery. During the morning assessment the nurse identifies a new finding of S3 heart sound. The lung sounds are clear without the presence of crackles. The nurse determines that these findings are:

   A. Normal for a patient with this cardiac history

   B. An indication of volume overload and CHF

   C. Early closure of the mitral and tricuspid valves

   D. A normal sound heard in late diastole

2. The nurse is caring for a client who has a history of rheumatic heart disease affecting the mitral valve. During the assessment of this client's heart sounds, the nurse would best hear murmurs of the mitral valve by listening in what part of the client's chest?

   A. Third intercostal space to the right of the sternum

   B. Third intercostal space to the left of the sternum

   C. Fifth intercostal space to the left of the sternum

   D. Fifth intercostal space at the apex

3. The nurse is caring for an 82-year-old client who develops a temperature of 100°F and a cough. The client's respirations are 20 and the pulse oximetry reading is 96% on room air. This morning's chest x-ray report states lungs are clear. During the morning assessment, there are bronchial breath sounds in the right lung field. Which of the following nursing interventions would the nurse take?

   A. Contact the client's physician to report assessment findings

   B. Continue to monitor the client's temperature

   C. Administer Tylenol to treat the patient's temperature

   D. Ask the patient to cough to determine if the bronchial breath sounds will clear

4. During the morning assessment of lung sounds of a client diagnosed with pneumonia, the nurse notes a leathery sound in the right lung fields. The nurse determines this finding to indicate:

   A. Increased peribronchial lymphatics causing airway compression

   B. Congestion of the lung fields from the pneumonia infiltrate

   C. Progression of the pneumonia to the pleura

   D. A normal finding in a client with pneumonia

5. The nurse in the emergency department is assessing a 56-year-old client who was an unrestrained driver in a motor vehicle accident. The client reports hitting the steering wheel on impact and complains of pain in the left chest and under his left arm. The client's respirations are shallow at 28/min and heart rate at 104/minute. Auscultation of breath sounds is diminished on the left lung fields and increased in the right lung fields. The nurse would respond initially to these findings by:

A. Starting two large bore IVs

B. Performing an EKG

C. Maintaining the client's airway and administering oxygen

D. Preparing for chest tube insertion

6. During auscultation of the chest of a client with an exacerbation of asthma the nurse notices the absence of wheezing and a quiet chest. The nurse interprets this to indicate the:

A. Airway is clear

B. Client may need intubation

C. Asthma is resolved

D. Expiratory phase of respiration is shortened

7. The nurse completed an assessment of the breath sounds of a client with a diagnosis of chronic obstructive pulmonary disease (COPD). The nurse notes rhonchi and occasional wheezing. To further assess airflow obstruction the nurse would:

A. Listen with the diaphragm of the stethoscope while asking the patient to cough

B. Listen with the bell of the stethoscope over the sternal notch at the base of the neck while asking the client to take a deep breath and blow out as fast as possible

C. Listen with the diaphragm of the stethoscope while asking the client to say the letter "E" and noting the sound to decrease in resonance

D. Listen for increased resonance to whispered words

8. The nurse has just completed the extubation of a client. Immediately following this procedure, the nurse notes a wheeze during inspiration. The nurse would contact the physician and:

A. Prepare for reintubation

B. Elevate the head of the bed

C. Administer high-flow oxygen

D. Obtain an order for an anti-inflammatory agent

9. The nurse auscultates an S4 during the assessment of a client's heart sounds. The nurse would consider this finding innocent unless it is associated with what additional assessment data indicating it is associated with a pathologic state?

A. Hematocrit of 35%

B. Blood pressure of 180/120

C. Client age of 82

D. Decreased Thyroxine (T4)

10. The nurse notes a split of S2 during the assessment of heart sounds. The nurse would consider this an abnormal finding to report to the physician when it is:

A. During inspiration in the adult

B. During expiration in children in the supine position

C. In an infant at the left sternal border

D. Prolonged or fixed

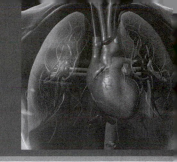

ANSWERS TO WORKBOOK EXERCISES

CHAPTER 1 – INTRODUCTION

Exercise 1 - Heart Anatomy and Auscultatory Sites

1. Atrioventricular
2. Semilunar
3. Atrioventricular
4. Semilunar
5. Atrioventricular
6. Semilunar

Exercise 2 - Valvular Disease and Murmur Location

Valve	Systolic Murmur	Diastolic Murmur
Aortic	Aortic stenosis	Aortic insufficiency
Pulmonic	Pulmonary stenosis	Pulmonary insufficiency
Mitral	Mitral insufficiency	Mitral stenosis
Tricuspid	Tricuspid insufficiency	Tricuspid stenosis

Exercise 3 - Auscultatory Sites

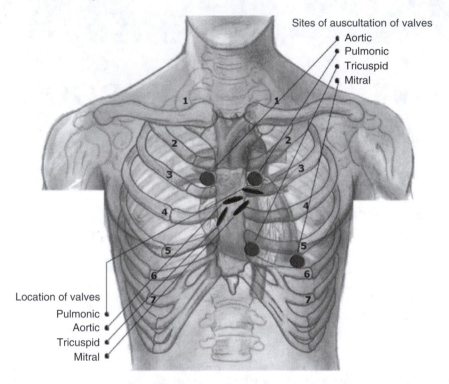

Sites of auscultation of valves
- Aortic
- Pulmonic
- Tricuspid
- Mitral

Location of valves
- Pulmonic
- Aortic
- Tricuspid
- Mitral

Exercise 4 - Murmur Mechanism Guide—Matching

Answers:

Aortic stenosis   Turbulence caused by the flow of blood through a narrowed semilunar valve that radiates to the carotids

Pulmonic regurgitation   Heard in the left sternal border, it results from backflow of the semilunar valve carrying unoxygenated blood

Normal diastole   Atrioventricular valves open and semilunar valves closed

Patent ductus arteriosis   A continual connection between the aorta and pulmonary artery causing a pressure differential that results in continuous turbulence and a systolic murmur

Ventricular septal defect   Flow of blood from a higher pressure chamber to the lower pressure; murmur is holosystolic

Mitral stenosis   Turbulence caused by a narrowed valve causing a diastolic murmur

Aortic insufficiency   Caused by backflow of oxygenated blood during diastole

Mitral regurgitation   Systolic murmur that may radiate to the axilla

Atrial septal defect   Mid-diastolic rumble due to increased blood flow through the tricuspid valve

Normal systole   Atrioventricular valves closed, semilunar valves open

Tricuspid regurgitation   Turbulent blood flow that the murmur may radiate to the apex via papillary muscles

Pulmonic stenosis   Narrowed valve with the murmur heard at the second intercostal space to the left of the sternal border

Tricuspid stenosis   Narrowed atrioventricular valve heard at the fifth intercostal space to the left of the sternal border

Exercise 5 - Assessing Repiratory Function

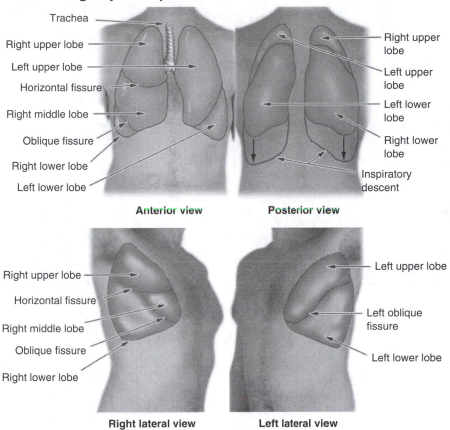

Exercise 6 - Ascultatory Sites for Lung Sounds

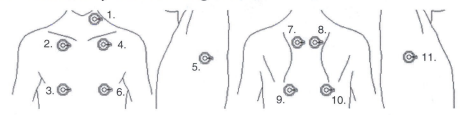

1. Trachea
2. Right upper lobe
3. Right middle lobe
4. Left upper lobe
5. Left lower lobe
6. Left lower lobe
7. Left upper lobe
8. Right upper lobe

9. Left lower lobe
10. Right lower lobe
11. Right lower lobe

Exercise 7 - Physical Assessment of the Respiratory System

1. The purpose of percussion is to cause the underlying tissue to vibrate and produce sound. The sound or note produced depends on the density of the underlying tissues.

2. Percussion over normal lung results in a note that is higher pitched or more resonant than percussion over denser tissue, such as the liver or the heart, which results in a dull note.

3. Resonance Table:

Type of Resonance	Source of Sounds	Underlying Disease Pathology
Normal Resonance	Heard over most of chest, the resonance is a reflection of air in the lung cavities	No underlying pathology
Hyperresonance	Tympanic or drumlike sound, this resonance is present when the density of tissue under the percussing finger is less dense than normal	Collapsed lung with a pneumothorax or advanced stages of emphysema
Decreased Resonance	Dull or flat sound, this resonance is present when the tissue under the percussing finger is more dense than normal	Normal: Over the heart Abnormal: Pneumonia with consolidation or pleural effusion

4. A—Dull
   B—Dull
   C—Liver
   D—Resonance
   E—Dull
   F—High level spinal cord injury, drug or anesthetic effect, neuromuscular diseases such as Guillain-Barré, Myasthenia Gravis, or Amyotrophic Lateral Sclerosis

CHAPTER 2 – COMMON HEART SOUNDS

Exercise 1 - Common Heart Sound Review

Common Heart Sound Review—Matching
Answers:

<u>Closure of mitral and tricuspid valves</u>   Start of systole

<u>Rising phase of pulse</u>   S1 sound corresponds with this phase of the pulse

<u>Declining phase of pulse</u>   S2 sound corresponds with this phase of the pulse

<u>Bradycardia</u>   Heart rate below normal values

<u>Ventricular ejection (systole)</u>   Time between the first and second heart sound

<u>Children age 1–10 years heart rates</u>   70–120 beats/minute

<u>Closure of aortic and pulmonic valves</u>   End of systole

<u>Athlete heart rates</u>   40–60 beats/minute

<u>Tachycardia</u>   Rate above normal values

<u>Infant heart rates</u>   100–160 beats/minute

<u>Lub</u>   First heart sound

<u>Children age 10 years and older heart rates</u>   60–100 beats/minute

<u>Ventricular filling (diastole)</u>   Time between the second heart sound and the following first heart sound

<u>Dub</u>   Second heart sound

Exercise 2 - Differentiating S3 and S4

Heart Sound	Associated Heart Process	Normal Characteristics	Pathologic Characteristics	Cadence Word Clue
S3	Early diastolic filling	Heard more often in children than adults Waxes and wanes May disappear when the patient sits up	Higher pitch Louder More constant sound Associated with volume overload and left ventricular systolic dysfunction	"Ken-tu-cky"
S4	Late diastolic, atrial filling	No typical characteristics	Seen in uncontrolled hypertension	"Ten-nes-see"

Exercise 3 - Rate, Rhythm, and Splitting of Heart Sounds

1. Answer: During inspiration the diaphragm contracts moving inferiorly toward the abdomen. This causes an *increase* in intra-abdominal pressure and decrease in intrathoracic pressure. The result causes an *increase* in venous return.

2. With the increase in venous return, there is a corresponding increase in stroke volume and heart rate during inspiration and a slowing down during expiration.

3. There are many types of heart dysrhythmias that may cause an irregular heart rate. One of the most common is atrial fibrillation. This is a condition where the atria fibrillate instead of contracting rhythmically with the cardiac cycle. The ventricles will respond by contracting at an irregular rate, causing the irregularity of the heart rate. Heart blocks, premature contractions, and other atrial and ventricular dysrhythmias may cause irregular heart rates.

   One method to identify the source of the irregularity is to take the pulse and listen to the heart rate for 1 full minute to determine the pattern and if it is associated with the respiratory cycle. Another method would be to place the client on a cardiac monitor which will precisely identify an abnormal cardiac rhythm.

4. Mitral and tricuspid valves close at different times.

5. Aortic and pulmonic valves close at different times.

6. During inspiration the diaphragm contracts, moving inferiorly toward the abdomen. This causes an *increase* in intra-abdominal pressure and decrease in intrathoracic pressure. The result causes an *increase* in venous return. This increase in blood may take the right ventricle longer to pump blood through the pulmonary artery. Consequently, the pulmonic valve closure will be delayed compared to the aortic valve closure, causing a split of S2.

Exercise 4 - Characteristics of Splitting of S2

Splitting of S2	Cause	Effect on the Heart Valves
Normal	Inspiration and increased venous return on the right heart	Pulmonic closure is delayed.
Mild Paradoxical	Inspiration and increased venous return on the right heart	Pulmonic closure is delayed but there is a narrowing of the S2 split with inspiration.
Advanced Paradoxical	Prolonged left ventricular ejection time Severe aortic stenosis Left ventricular outflow obstruction Left ventricular overload (patent ductus arteriosus) Conduction abnormalities that cause prolonged left ventricular ejection (left bundle branch block, premature ventricular contractions, Wolf-Parkinson-White syndrome)	Aortic valve closes later than the pulmonic valve. Normally the pulmonic valve closes first, then the aortic valve. In this condition, it is reversed.

Exercise 5 - Heart Murmurs

1.

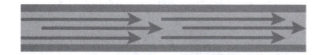

Cause: Increased flow through a normal structure

Clinical conditions in which murmur can occur: Anemia causing an aortic systolic murmur

2.

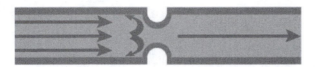

Cause: Stenosis causing obstruction to flow

Clinical conditions in which murmur can occur: Mitral and aortic stenosis

3.

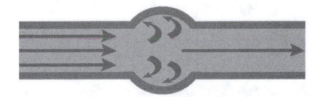

Cause: Flow into a dilated chamber; vortex formation as blood flows from a narrower to a larger chamber

Clinical conditions in which murmur can occur: Aortic valve is normal in size and aorta is dilated

4.

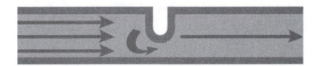

Cause: Membrane that vibrates

Clinical conditions in which murmur can occur: Papillary muscle rupture

5.

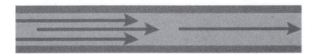

Cause: Flow of blood from a high pressure to a low pressure

Clinical conditions in which murmur can occur: Ventricular septal defects

Exercise 6 - Murmur Timing

1. Systolic
2. Diastolic
3. Increased heart rates. Normally systole is short and diastole is longer. The duration of systole may become almost the same as the duration of diastole, making it hard to distinguish systole and diastole.

4. ■ Observing apex movement
   ■ Feeling the pulse
   ■ Watching the EKG

5. Continuous

6. Murmurs of both systolic and diastolic components. Unlike continuous murmurs, there is a distinct silence between the systolic and diastolic phases.

Exercise 7 - Murmur Location and Radiation

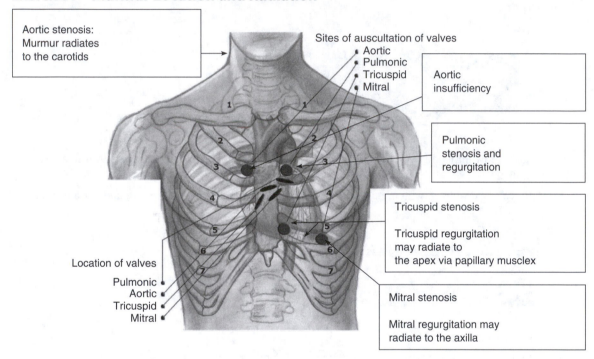

Exercise 8 - Murmur Grading—Matching

Answers:

Grade 4   Loud murmur; a thrill may be present

Grade 1   Faint murmur that can only be heard after a few seconds

Grade 6   Loud murmur that can be heard with the chest piece just removed from and not touching the skin; a thrill is present

Grade 2   Faint murmur that is heard immediately

Grade 5   Loud murmur that can be heard if only the edge of the stethoscope is in contact with the skin; a thrill is present

Grade 3   Moderate murmur intensity

Exercise 9 - Murmur Shape

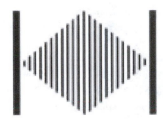

Crescendo/Decrescendo—low intensity, steady increase in intensity with a steady decrease in intensity

1. Stenotic valves
2. Diamond shaped murmurs, ejection type murmurs

Holosystolic—present throughout systole and are uniform in intensity

1. Pansystolic

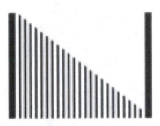

Decrescendo—starts at high intensity and decreases in intensity

1. Diastolic murmurs of aortic and pulmonic regurgitation.
2. With aortic and pulmonic regurgitation, there is backflow of blood from a valve that doesn't close completely. The turbulence begins with S2 and declines as the ventricle fills and the pressure difference between the artery and ventricle decreases. With mitral and tricuspid stenosis, a decrescendo murmur is heard as blood flows into a ventricle through a narrowed valve.

Exercise 10 - Systolic and Diastolic Murmur Timing

Type of Murmur	Timing	Other Defining Characteristics
Early Systolic	First third of systole	
Mid Systolic	Shortly after S1	Crescendo/decrescendo As ejection increases the murmur gets louder then diminishes as ejection decreases
Late Systolic	Starts well after ejection and ends before S2	Soft and high pitched Ischemia or infarction of the mitral papillary muscles Prolapse of mitral valve leaflets into the left atrium
Early Diastolic	Shortly after S2	In the presence of pulmonic regurgitation this murmur may be associated with pulmonary hypertension
Mid Diastolic	Occurs between S2 and S1	Soft and difficult to hear Originates from the mitral and tricuspid valves
Late Diastolic	Just prior to S1 called presystolic or protosystolic	Usually due to mitral and tricuspid stenosis

Exercise 11 - Systolic Murmur Pitch

1. There is a higher pressure gradient during systole as blood flows through a stenotic aortic valve, causing a louder sound. The pressure gradient is less during diastole when blood flows through a stenotic mitral valve.

Exercise 12, 13, 14 and 15 (Draw images or copy images from manuscript)

Figure 2-1

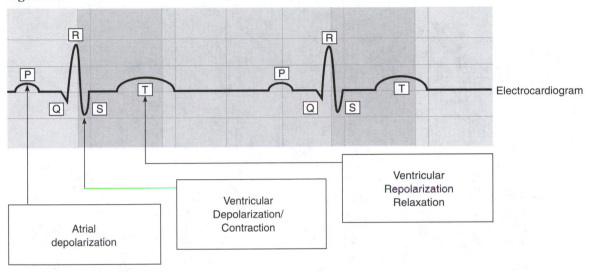

Figure 2-2

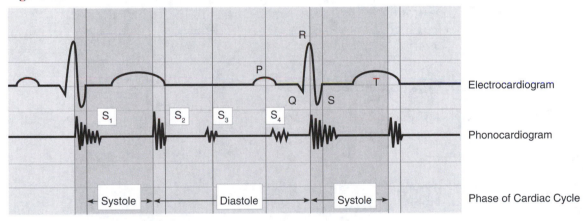

Figure 2-3

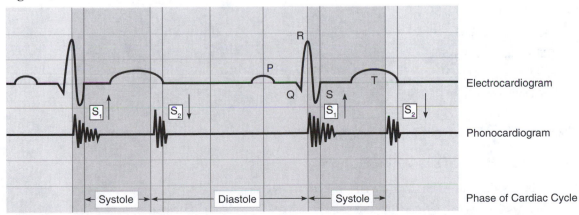

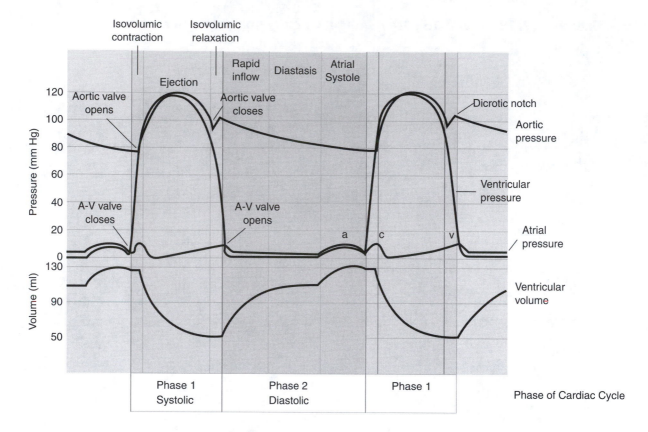

Exercise 16 - Phase 1 of the Cardiac Cycle

Fill-in-the-Blanks

1. Close
2. Contraction, systolic
3. QRS
4. Upswing

Exercise 17 - Phase 2 of the Cardiac Cycle

Fill-in-the-Blanks

1. Close, second
2. Relaxation, diastolic
3. T wave
4. Downswing

CHAPTER 3 – COMMON LUNG SOUNDS

Exercise 1 - Normal Breathing Sounds

1. Normal: Occur when there are no respiratory problems
2. Adventitious: Abnormal, indicating the existence of a pathologic state

3.

____V____ Resemble wind moving through trees, causing leaves to rustle

____B____ Heard over large airways

____B____ Louder during expiration

____B____ Air being blown through a cardboard roll

____B____ Heard over the trachea or in the midline of the upper anterior chest

____B____ Heard over the right upper anterior chest and on the back between the scapulae, both to the right and left of the sternum

____V____ Heard over small airways of the chest

____B____ When heard at the base of the lungs, are considered abnormal

____B____ Commonly heard when lung tissue becomes solid

____B____ Pneumonia, or any situation in which the alveoli and the small airways are filled with fluid, will produce these breath sounds in abnormal locations

____B____ Heard louder on expiration than inspiration

____V____ Heard louder on inspiration than expiration

Exercise 2 - Sound Visualization

1. **Expanded:** The time or x axis is stretched out so that the details of the acoustic phenomenon can be examined

   Unexpanded: The overall view of the acoustic characteristic in real time

2. The amplitude–versus–time plots will reveal visually distinct patterns not readily seen in plots at conventional speeds

Exercise 3 – Adventitious Sounds

Adventitious Sound	Description	Acoustic Characteristic	Potential Sources of Abnormal Sound	Discontinuous vs. Continuous
Fine Crackles	Cracking noise when salt is heated on a frying pan Sound when wood burns	High pitch explosive sound Less intense Shorter duration	Sudden opening of airways Fluid in the airways	Discontinuous
Coarse Crackles	Crackling noise when salt is heated on a frying pan Sound when wood burns	Louder Slightly longer in duration Lower pitch bubbling sound	Sudden opening of airways Fluid in the airways	Discontinuous
Wheezes	Musical quality Sinusoidal pattern	High pitch Whistling or sibilant sound	Airway narrowing and bronchospasm Airway edema secretions Endobronchial tumors Extrinsic compression of an airway In CHF due to increased fluid in peribronchia lymphatics that cause airway compression	Continuous
Squawks	Short wheezes Brief squeaky sounds	Brief duration	Bird fanciers disease Hypersensitivity pneumonitis and pneumonia Heard when alveolitis is present (e.g., pneumonia)	Discontinuous
Rhonchi	Snoring quality Usually clear with coughing	Low pitch	Airway secretions Airway narrowing	Continuous

Pleural Rub	Leathery or grating sound	Discontinuous—may sound like fine crackles Heard on inspiration and expiration	Diseases involving the surface of pleura such as pleuritis or pneumonia that has spread from the lung tissue to the pleural space	Discontinuous and continuous
Stridor	Sounds like a wheezing noise Can be heard with or without a stethoscope Can observe use of accessory muscles of respiration during inspiration and retraction of supraclavicular fossae	Prominent during *inspiration* Similar to a wheeze Loudest over mouth, neck, and upper trachea	Upper airway obstruction Note or observe: Food in mouth or evidence of foreign body aspirate Check neck for masses, scars, and tracheal deviation Check skin for hives that may indicate angioneurotic edema of the glottis Heard immediately after extubation; may require reintubation	Continuous

Exercise 4 - Approach to the Patient

1. Breathe deeply, keeping mouth open
2. Stop the exam and ask the patient to hold his or her breath for a moment
3. Right upper lobe posteriorly
4. Diaphragm
5. Hair
6. Wet the chest wall and press more firmly against the chest wall with the stethoscope
7. Lung bases during expiration

CHAPTER 4 – LUNG SOUND PATTERNS

Exercise 1 - Lung Sound Analyzer

Fill-in-the-Blank

1. Stethograph or STG
2. Crackles and wheezes

Exercise 2 - Lung Sounds and Disease

Matching
Answers:

COPD   Decreased, end-expiratory wheezing; rhonchi that clear with coughing and basilar crackles

Congestive heart failure   Numerous crackles over the chest from bases to apices

Bronchiectasis   Crackles are common over affected area, often over posterior bases, present for years without changing

Pneumonia   Crackles over affected region, dullness to percussion, decreased breath sounds and bronchial breathing

Pneumothorax   Absence of breath sounds over affected area

Interstitial fibrosis   Fine crackles, squawks, and short wheezes

Asthma   Cardinal feature is wheezing

Tuberculosis   Abnormal lung sounds heard in upper half of chest, inspiratory crackles, amphoric or cavernous sounds

Exercise 3 - Changes in Lung Sound Pattern

True and False

1. False
2. False
3. True
4. True
5. False
6. False

NCLEX® CERTIFICATION QUESTIONS—ANSWERS AND RATIONALES

1. Answer: B
Rationale: S3 is a sign of a pathologic process of volume overload that will cause early diastolic filling. Many patients with congestive heart failure present with no crackles and an S3 during assessment. S3 is not a normal finding with a client with a history of cardiac disease. The S3 is heard just following S2, the closure of the aortic and pulmonic valves, giving it a rhythmic gallop sound of Ken-tu-cky. It is heard in early diastole, not late diastole.

    Nursing Process: Assessment
    Category of Client Need: Physiologic integrity
    Cognitive Level: Analysis

2. Answer: D
Rationale: D is the location for auscultation of the mitral valve. Murmurs of the mitral valve may also be heard in the axillary region. A is the location for the aortic valve, B is the location for the pulmonic valve, and C is the location for the tricuspid valve.

    Nursing Process: Assessment
    Category of Client Need: Physiologic integrity
    Cognitive Level: Analysis

3. Answer: A

Rationale: Bronchial breath sounds in the lung field of the smaller airways is a sign of a disease process that makes the lung tissue solid. It is not normal to hear bronchial breath sounds in the smaller airways. An early clinical finding in clients with a fever and cough is bronchial breath sounds in the smaller airways, indicating the presence of pneumonia up to 1 day before the chest x-ray shows any clear-cut evidence of the disease. While the physician makes the final clinical diagnosis, it is the nurses' role to inform the physician of these key assessment findings that indicate the presence of pneumonia. Monitoring and treating the temperature are good interventions but delay in obtaining valuable treatment for this client's clinical condition. Abnormal bronchial breath sounds clear when there is resolution of the disease. Rhonchi are abnormal breath sounds that will characteristically clear with coughing.

    Nursing Process: Implementation
    Category of Client Need: Physiologic integrity
    Cognitive Level: Application

4. Answer: C

Rationale: When the pleura are inflamed from an infectious process, it will present a sound during the breathing that resembles leather rubbing together. This is called a pleural rub. A common source for this sound is the progression of pneumonia into the pleura and is never a normal finding. With increased peribronchial lymphatics airway compression occurs and presents with a wheezing sound in the presence of congestive heart failure. Congestion of the lung fields with pneumonia will present a crackle sound.

    Nursing Process: Assessment
    Category of Client Need: Physiologic integrity
    Cognitive Level: Analysis

5. Answer: C

Rationale: The client's assessment data are indicative of hypoxia and a pneumothorax. Lung sounds are often diminished or absent in the affected lung field with an increase on the opposite side of the chest. A pneumothorax will result in hypoxia due to the collapsing of the lung. Therefore, the nurse's initial actions are to protect an open airway and administer oxygen to decrease hypoxia. The client's assessment data are indicative of a pneumothorax which must be confirmed with a chest x-ray prior to chest tube insertion. Starting IVs, performing an EKG, and preparing for chest tube insertion must be done after the client's airway is maintained and hypoxia is addressed.

    Nursing Process: Implementation
    Category of Client Need: Physiologic integrity
    Cognitive Level: Application

6. Answer: B

Rationale: A quiet chest in a known asthmatic client is an ominous finding that only occurs for a brief period prior to his or her recovery, intubation, or death. It is an indicator of no air movement, not resolution of the asthma or clearing of the airway. Option D is incorrect because the expiratory phase in an asthmatic is longer, not shorter.

    Nursing Process: Assessment
    Category of Client Need: Physiologic integrity
    Cognitive Level: Analysis

7. Answer: B

Rationale: The technique of listening with the bell of the stethoscope and asking the patient to take a deep breath and blow out is used to time the audible expiratory phase to calculate the FEV1/FVC ratio. This is a simple bedside technique used with COPD patients to detect airflow obstruction. The technique in option A is a method to determine if rhonchi clear with coughing. Options C and D are assessment techniques used to determine vocal resonance and lung consolidation, and may be present in emphysema. Vocal resonance with the client saying "E" will change to a broad "A" sound and whispered words will decrease in resonance, not increase.

Nursing Process: Assessment
Category of Client Need: Physiologic integrity
Cognitive Level: Analysis

8. Answer: A
Rationale: An inspiratory wheeze is characteristic of upper airway obstruction; when it occurs immediately after extubation it may indicate the need for reintubation. While elevating the head of the bed and giving oxygen may facilitate respiration and decrease hypoxia, if the airway is obstructed, these interventions would be futile. Anti-inflammatory agents are used to decrease airway edema but take time to reach a therapeutic effect. In this client, airway obstruction and hypoxia are critical to survival and need to be addressed immediately.

Nursing Process: Implementation
Category of Client Need: Physiologic integrity
Cognitive Level: Application

9. Answer: B
Rationale: S4 is an abnormal finding in the presence of uncontrolled hypertension and other pathologic states such as coronary artery disease, profound anemia, pregnancy, and thyrotoxicosis. The hematocrit level is within normal values and S4 is often normal in the elderly client. The decreased Thyroxine level is seen in hypothyroidism and elevated in hyperthyroidism, which is the pathologic state present with thyrotoxicosis.

Nursing Process: Assessment
Category of Client Need: Physiologic integrity
Cognitive Level: Analysis

10. Answer: D
Rationale: Splitting occurs normally when associated with respiration. It is a result of an increase in abdominal pressure and a corresponding decrease of intrathoracic pressure that leads to increased venous return from the systemic circulation of the right heart. It takes a little longer for the right ventricle to pump the increased amount of blood. Consequently, the pulmonic valve closure is delayed compared to the aortic valve closure. The splitting occurs in children during expiration when in a supine position and is found in infants at the left sternal border. When the split of S2 is fixed or prolonged, this is a result of a pathologic process such as a delay in activation of contraction, delay in emptying of the right ventricle, large atrial septal defects, or right ventricular failure.

Nursing Process: Assessment
Category of Client Need: Physiologic integrity
Cognitive Level: Analysis

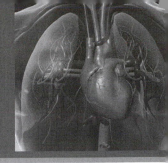

GLOSSARY

The terms listed in this glossary are found in the materials provided in this workbook, the *A Simplified Introduction to Heart and Lung Sounds for Nurses* CD, and the articles and books from the reference list. They are selected to give you a comprehensive list of the common terms used in this area of nursing and medicine.

Ankylosing spondylitis: Genetically based disease (HLA B27 antigen positive) characterized by fusion of the vertebral bodies ("bamboo spine") joint inflammation and dilatation of the aortic root.

Asthma: Disease of the respiratory system that involves inflammation of the bronchial tubes which causes cough, wheeze, dyspnea, and varying degrees of reversible airflow obstruction. This inflammatory disorder, typically due to an allergic reaction, causes the airways to narrow, leading to difficulty breathing.

Atrial myxoma: Benign tumor of the atrium often causing valvular obstruction or embolic phenomenon.

Bioprosthetic valve: Artificial valve constructed from biological tissue.

Bronchial sounds (same as tracheal sounds): Heard on the chest at sites which are close to large airways. In contrast to vesicular sounds, they are relatively louder in expiration than inspiration. They have a tubular or hollow quality similar to air being blown through a tube.

Bronchiectasis: This disorder is characterized by abnormal destruction and dilation of bronchi or bronchioles. It can be caused by a chronic inflammatory or degenerative condition of one or more bronchi or bronchioles marked by dilatation and loss of elasticity of the wall. It is commonly associated with chronic, productive cough.

Carcinoid heart disease: Thickening of the heart valves (right side more commonly), often with marked regurgitation associated with a metastatic carcinoid tumor. (Carcinoid is of a chromaffin cell origin, usually originating in the small bowel.)

Cardiomegaly: Type of progressive heart disease in which the heart is abnormally enlarged, thickened, and stiffened. As a result, the hearts' ability to pump blood is weakened, often causing heart failure and the backup of blood into the lungs.

CHF (congestive heart failure): Heart failure in which the heart is unable to maintain an adequate circulation of blood in the tissues of the body or to pump out the blood returned to it by the venous circulation.

Chordae tendinae: A thin supporting structure of the atrioventricular valves connecting the leaflets to the papillary muscles.

Chronic bronchitis: The American Thoracic Society defines chronic bronchitis "as a clinical disorder characterized by excessive mucus secretions manifested by chronic or productive cough. On most days for a minimum of 3 months of the year and for not less than two successive years." Unfortunately, other disorders with similar manifestations must be excluded, such as bronchiectasis, tuberculosis, and lung abscess. Patients with predominant asthma or emphysema may fit this distinction. Many patients with pathological or physiological hallmarks of chronic bronchitis may not qualify under this definition; that is, they do not cough.

Coarse crackles (also known as coarse rales): Intermittent explosive sounds that have been described as being similar to the crackling sound heard as wood burns. On auscultation coarse crackles are in general lower pitched (less than 400 Hz), less intense, and of longer duration than fine crackles.

COPD (chronic obstructive pulmonary disease): A condition in which there is a fixed and progressive obstruction to airflow. COPD is a designated label for a group of lung diseases. The two diseases that generally are associated with COPD are chronic bronchitis and emphysema. Chronic obstructive pulmonary disease (COPD) refers to a group of disorders that have in common persistent airflow obstruction. Pathologically, chronic bronchitis and emphysema are distinct, bronchitis being limited to the airways and emphysema to the pulmonary parenchyma. From a clinical point of view, the distinction between bronchitis and emphysema is difficult. Both processes may be present in the same patient and both are characterized by expiratory flow obstruction. Furthermore, the patients with both processes often present with the same symptom; namely, dyspnea on exertion. Both may have airway hyperreactivity. The situation is further complicated by the fact that patients with either disease may have the airway hyperreactivity as is seen in asthma. Consequently, lumping these conditions into this single label, COPD, is useful.

Crackle family: Crackles, which are explosive sounds associated with an airway opening, can often be detected by multiple microphones on the chest. Crackles occurring within 5 ms likely represent the same event of airway opening and are called a crackle family. The crackle with highest deflection is called the mother crackle and the corresponding deflections at other channels are termed daughter crackles. As a rule of thumb crackles in patients with CHF and pneumonia are transmitted over an area about the size of the palm.

Crackle rate: The number of crackles per breath or the number of crackles per second. A normal person may have up to two crackles per breath. Very high crackle rates are found in interstitial fibrosis.

Ebstein's anomaly: Congenital anomaly characterized by inferior displacement of the tricuspid valve resulting in a small "true" right ventricle inferior to the tricuspid valve and an "atrialized" component of the right ventricle along with the true right atrium superior to the valve.

Eisenmenger's physiology: Reversal of flow through a cardiac defect from *L to R* to *R to L* because of an increase in right-sided pressures secondary to marked pulmonary hypertension. Pulmonary hypertension, in turn, is due to increased peripheral pulmonary vascular impedance.

Emphysema: The American Thoracic Society defines emphysema as an anatomical alteration of the lung characterized by an abnormal enlargement of the air spaces distal to the nonrespiratory bronchioles accompanied by destructive changes of the alveolar walls.

Endocarditis: Inflammation of the valvular leaflets often secondary to a bacterial infection. Noninfectious causes such as lupus are less common.

FEV1:   Forced expiratory volume is the amount of air that the patient can exhale in one second.

Fine crackles (also known as fine rales):   Intermittent explosive sounds that have been described as being similar to the crackling sound heard as wood burns. On auscultation fine crackles are in general higher pitched (over 400 Hz), less intense, and of shorter duration than coarse crackles.

First degree AV block: Prolongation of conduction time through the atria or through the AV node manifesting as a prolonged PR interval on the surface electrocardiogram.

FVC: Forced vital capacity is the total amount of air that the patient can exhale after a deep inspiration.

Gallavardin phenomenon: Radiation of the aortic stenosis murmur to the apex (most commonly seen in the elderly).

Hepatojugular reflux: An increased pressure on the liver, which causes an increased central venous pressure.

Hepatomegaly: Enlarged liver; common in right heart failure patients.

Homograft: Artificial valve consisting of a transplanted biological valve from the same species as the recipient.

Jugular venous distention: Seen as a bulging neck vein when the right ventricle fails to pump blood through pulmonary circulation, which in turn backs up into the vein.

Lupus: Collagen vascular disease associated with autoantibodies to various organs. May be associated with the formation of noninfectious endocarditis.

Marfan's syndrome: Syndrome characterized by a connective tissue defect resulting in a tendency toward aortic dissection and/or expansion of the proximal aorta; is associated with mitral valve prolapse, hyperextendable joints, and lens dislocation. Patients are usually tall and thin with summation of the length from fingertip to fingertip of each arm when extended laterally exceeding or equaling their height.

Mucopolysaccharidosis: Deposition of abnormal fat and protein within the cardiac valve leaflets.

Noonan's syndrome: Characterized by impaired mental abilities, abnormal facies, hypertrophic cardiomyopathy, pulmonary or infundibular stenosis, peripheral pulmonary artery stenosis, patent ductus arteriosus, atrial septal defect, and tetralogy of Fallot.

Opening snap: High pitched presystolic sound associated with opening of a stiff atrioventricular valve.

Paradoxical splitting of the second heart sound: In its milder form paradoxical splitting of the S2 is associated with narrowing of a S2 split with inspiration. In the advanced form P2 of the second heart sound can appear before A2 (often due to prolonged flow through the aortic valve, causing a delay in closure).

Peripheral pitting edema: Swelling of the dependent body part, usually the ankles and feet. Commonly caused by chronic right heart failure where venous blood backs up, which increases the pressure gradient, causing leakage of fluid into the interstitial space.

Phen-fen: Weight loss drug associated with valvular abnormalities and/or pulmonary hypertension which is no longer available on the market.

Pleural rub: This sound has been compared to the sound made when two pieces of leather are rubbed together. It is believed to be caused by the surfaces of the pleura rubbing together. Normally these surfaces slide silently over each other. When they are inflamed the rubbing noise is made.

Pneumonia: Inflammation of the lung parenchyma that is usually caused by a microbial agent. In many cases, the term is modified to indicate a specific clinical setting, such as community-acquired pneumonia, nursing home pneumonia, pneumonia in the immunocompromised host, and aspiration pneumonia, among others. These terms are important because of differences in likely microbial agents, prognosis, and diagnostic evaluation. Other classifications are based on the tempo of the disease, such as acute, subacute, or chronic pneumonia. Classification may also be based on observations with radiographs or scans to characterize the changes as lobar pneumonia, bronchopneumonia, interstitial pneumonia, or lung abscess, and accompanying findings, such as hilar adenopathy, pleural fluid, or atelectasis.

Pneumothorax: A state in which air or other gas is present in the pleural cavity and which occurs spontaneously as a result of disease of the lung or puncture of the chest wall or is induced as a therapeutic measure (as in the treatment of tuberculosis).

Pulmonary vascular impedance: The resistance to flow existing within the blood vessels leading into or within the lung parenchyma.

Rhonchi (also known as sonorous rhonchi):   Also described as "continuous" sounds. They are lower in pitch than wheezes and have a snoring quality. The frequency is less than 200 Hz.

S3 or S4 gallop rhythm: Gallops are low frequency sounds that are associated with diastolic filling. The gallop associated with early diastolic filling is the S3 and may be heard pathologically in such states as volume overload and left ventricular systolic dysfunction. The S4 is a late diastolic sound and may be heard in such pathologic states as uncontrolled hypertension.

Sarcoidosis: Disorder characterized by abnormal formation of inflammatory masses or nodules (granulomas). Granulomas consist of certain granular white blood cells (modified macrophages or epithelioid cells). Granuloma formation most commonly affects the lungs, but can also affect the upper respiratory system, lymph nodes, skin, and eyes. The cause of sarcoidosis is not known.

Squawks: Short, inspiratory wheeze-like sounds that have been described in pneumonia, hypersensitivity pneumonitis, and other fibrotic disorders. Squawk duration is usually longer than 20 ms and shorter than 100 ms. The frequency is usually higher than 400 Hz.

Stridor: Characteristic feature of upper airway obstruction. Stridor is a continuous, high-pitched sound heard on auscultation, with or without a stethoscope, that is loudest over the mouth, neck, and upper trachea. The principal feature that distinguishes stridor from wheezing is that stridor is predominantly inspiratory.

Syphilis: Spirochete-based sexually transmitted disease which may be associated with inflammation, expansion, and/or dissection of the proximal aorta.

Tachycardia: Fast heartbeat, greater than 100 beats per minute in adults.

Tetralogy of Fallot: Congenital heart abnormality characterized by (1) pulmonary outflow tract obstruction such as pulmonic stenosis, (2) ventricular septal defect, (3) overriding aorta, and (4) right ventricular hypertrophy.

Time amplitude plot: Displays the waveform of sound. It is similar to a phonocardiogram. The amplitude is plotted on the y axis; time on the x axis. This may be done in real time or in the time expanded mode. The latter, by expanding the x axis, allows details of the waveform, such as the shape of crackles, to be more readily seen.

TLC: Total lung capacity is the maximum amount of air the lungs can hold when fully inflated.

Tuberculosis: Pulmonary tuberculosis is a parenchymal lung disease caused by *Mycobacterium tuberculosis*, slow-growing mycobacteria that thrive in areas of the body rich in blood and oxygen.

Unrelated crackles: Crackles that belong to different crackle families.

Valsalva: Physiologic maneuver in which intra-abdominal pressure is increased (usually by bearing down against a closed glottis) resulting in initial inhibition of right ventricular blood return followed by a rapid increase in return once abdominal pressure is released.

Vesicular sounds: Heard at sites that are at a distance from large airways. The vesicular sound is a soft sound that has been compared to that of wind blowing through trees. It is louder in inspiration than expiration.

Wheezes   (also known as sibilant rhonchi): Described as relatively "continuous" sounds as compared to crackles. They occur more often in expiration. They usually last for more than 200 milliseconds and have a musical quality. The frequency is greater than 200 Hz.

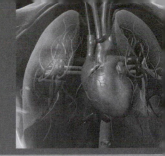

REFERENCES

Copstead, L. C., & Banaski, J. L. (2005). *Pathophysiology* (3rd ed.). St. Louis: Elsevier Inc.

Seidel, H. M., Ball, J. W., Dains, J. E., & Benedict, G. W. (2003). *Mosby's guide to physical examination* (5th ed.). St. Louis: Mosby.

Wagner, K. D., Johnson, K., & Kidd, P. S. (2005). *High acuity nursing* (4th ed.). Upper Saddle River, NJ: Prentice Hall.

Widmaier, E. P., Raff, H., Strang, K. T. *Vander, Sherman, & Luciano's* (2004). *Human physiology: The mechanism of body functions* (9th ed.). New York: McGraw-Hill.